Daniel Fast Juicing Bible

Disclaimer

Contents

Are you looking for a special juice diet with the power to cleanse your body and provide it with the nutrients that it requires? Well, what are you waiting for?

This report that we have prepared for you features exclusive Daniel Fast Juicing recipes which are considered to be highly beneficial for the human health. Going through it, you will find that the juices are made purely from fruits and vegetables which help give the human body the strength it needs to function in the best manner possible.

This book also includes individual nutritional facts for each juice that we have mentioned, so that you can get an idea of how much quantity of each nutrient you will be feeding to your body, if you prepare a certain juice for yourself. We are certain that you will love all the juice recipes and that you will incorporate as much of these in your daily life as you can.

These juices are bound to leave you refreshed and happy for the rest of your busy day. With a proper functioning body, there is no doubt that your day will be brighter and healthier.

Antioxidant Supreme

This delicious Antioxidant Supreme consists of fruits such as berries which have beneficial anti aging benefits. To make this juice, you will be needing one cup of fresh blueberries (either frozen or thawed), one cup of fresh strawberries (either frozen or thawed), two cups of chopped and peeled mango, and one fourth cup of water.

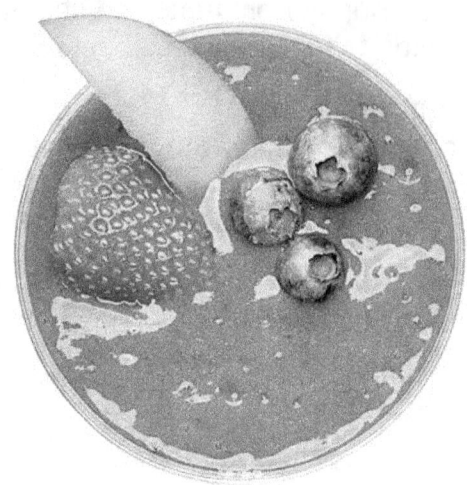

Nutritional Facts Per Serving:

Total Calories: 151

Fat: 1g

Protein: 2g

Carbohydrates: 38g

Fiber: 5g

Cholesterol: nil

Iron: 1mg

Sodium: 3mg

Calcium: 27mg

Apple Broccoli Blast

This juice can easily be made with two apples, which are cut into slices but unpeeled and cored, along with half a cup of broccoli florets and one cup of blueberries. Start by washing the ingredients well and then put the separated broccoli, blueberries and apples into the juicer. This will yield you two servings, which you can enjoy.

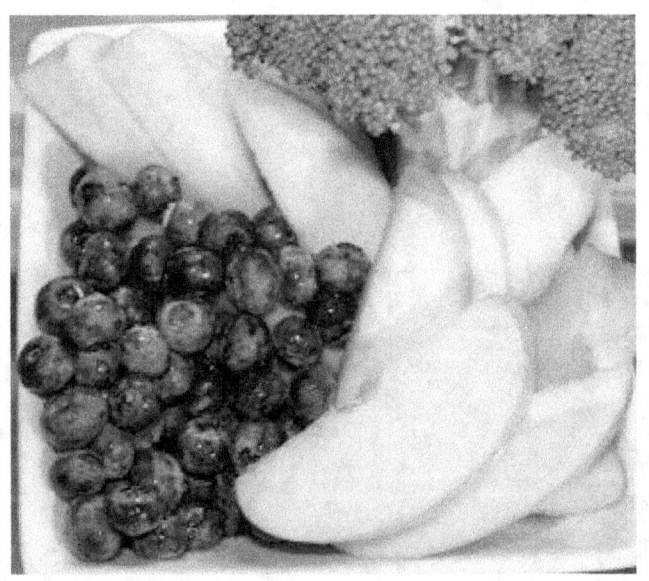

Nutrition Facts Per Serving:
Total Calories: 200

Fat: 2.09g

Protein: 13.04g

Carbohydrates: 57.68g

Fiber: 2.3g

Cholesterol: nil

Iron: 3.52mg

Sodium: 143mg

Calcium: 213mg

Beet Apple and Blackberry Juice

Beet juice is great for cleansing your blood. It consists of folate, vitamin C, iron, and manganese potassium. You can add blackberries, apples, and ginger to this juice for amazing taste and great color. To make this juice, you would need three small sized beets, two to three apples, eight oz. blackberries, and a half inch fresh ginger.

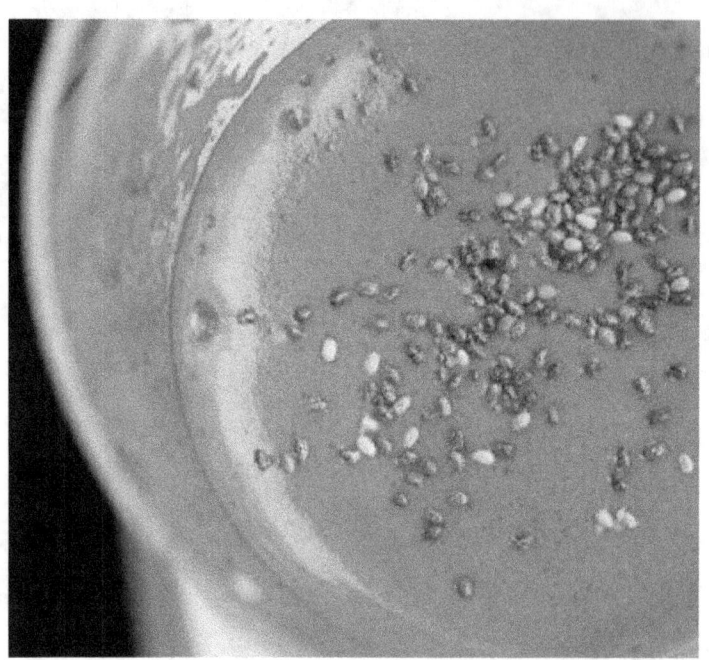

Nutrition Facts Per Serving:

Total Calories: 165

Fat: 0.96g

Protein: 4.17g

Carbohydrates: 51.61g

Fiber: 1.8g

Cholesterol: nil

Iron: 1.99mg

Sodium: 138mg

Calcium: 56mg

Beet Carrot Juice

Beet, along with carrot, makes a yummy combination. In addition, beet has many nutritional benefits such as helping in creating red blood cells, supplying body with iron, strengthening the liver, having anti cancer properties, and cleansing the stomach and intestines. This sweet and bright red juice can be made from one beet, the ends of which need to be removed and quartered, along with three to four carrots.

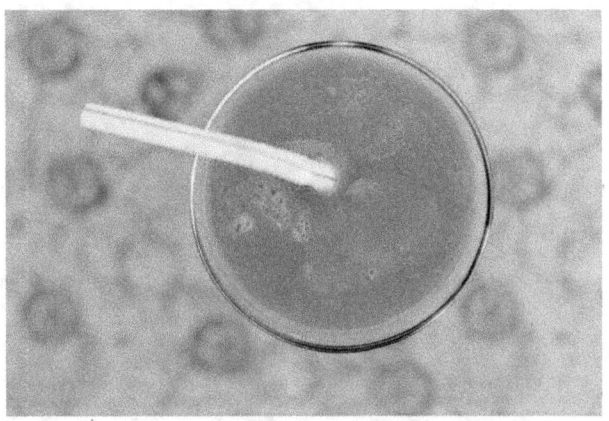

Nutrition Facts Per Serving:

Total Calories: 47

Fat: 0.31g

Protein: 1.76g

Carbohydrates: 14.07g

Fiber: 0.6g

Cholesterol: nil

Iron: 0.73mg

Sodium: 107mg

Calcium: 39mg

Beet Orange Juice

This juice requires you go obtain two oranges along with one beet, the ends of which are quartered and removed. You can mix these ingredients up in a juicer and serve. Orange helps add great taste to the juice along with health benefits, while beat already has a lot of amazing qualities.

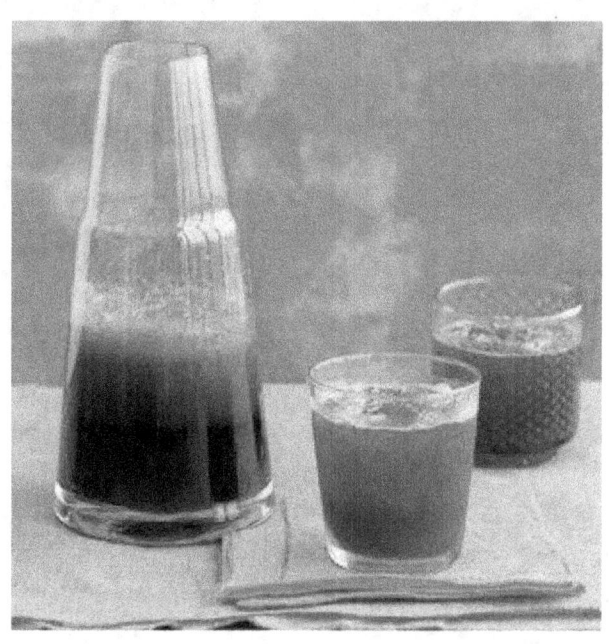

Nutritional Facts Per Serving:

Total Calories: 67

Fat: 0.25g

Protein: 2.11g

Carbohydrates: 20.29g

Fiber: 0.7g

Cholesterol: nil

Iron: 0.59mg

Sodium: 45mg

Calcium: 60mg

Beet Apple and Mint Juice

This juice helps to fight inflammation, detoxes your body, and helps to flush out toxins. The drink can easily be made with one small chopped beet, five chopped carrots, one cored and chopped apple, and one fourth cup of fresh mint sprigs.

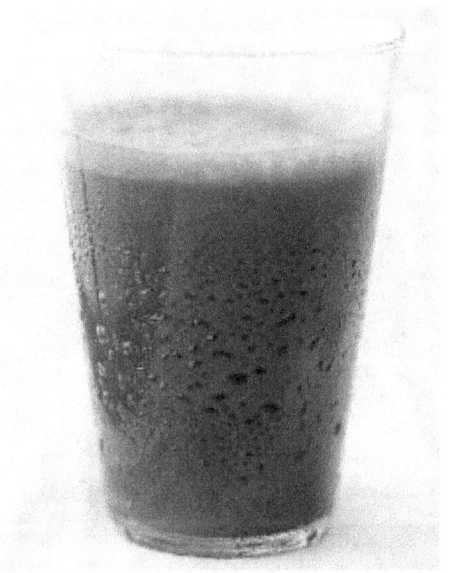

Nutritional Facts Per Serving:

Total Calories: 96

Fat: 0.47g

Protein: 2.57g

Carbohydrates: 29.49g

Fiber: 1g

Cholesterol: nil

Iron: 1.22mg

Sodium: 121mg

Calcium: 38mg

Blossoming Lotus Juice Aide

The Blossoming Lotus Juice Aide consists of simple ingredients which offer exquisite taste. To make this wonderful and sweet drink, you will need five large and cored Fuji apples, one (two inch) sliced and peeled fresh ginger, one medium sized lime, and seven large and sectioned sprigs cilantro.

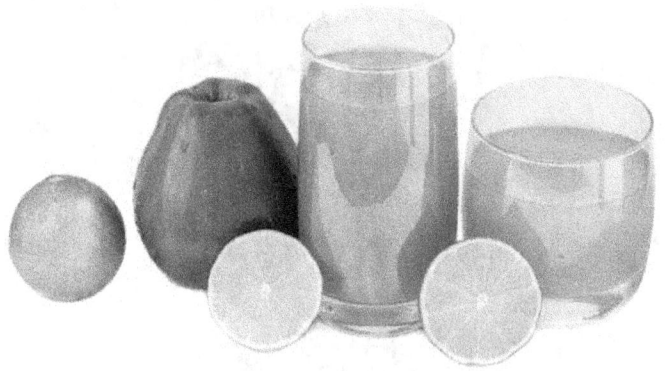

Nutritional Facts Per Serving:

Total Calories: 361

Fat: 1.57g

Protein: 2.77g

Carbohydrates: 115.90g

Fiber: 2.9g

Cholesterol: nil

Iron: 1.41mg

Sodium: 13mg

Calcium: 68mg

Carrot Apple Juice

This juice recipe is great for your health since it consists of four large carrots and two sweet apples. You can mix this to get an amazing refreshing drink.

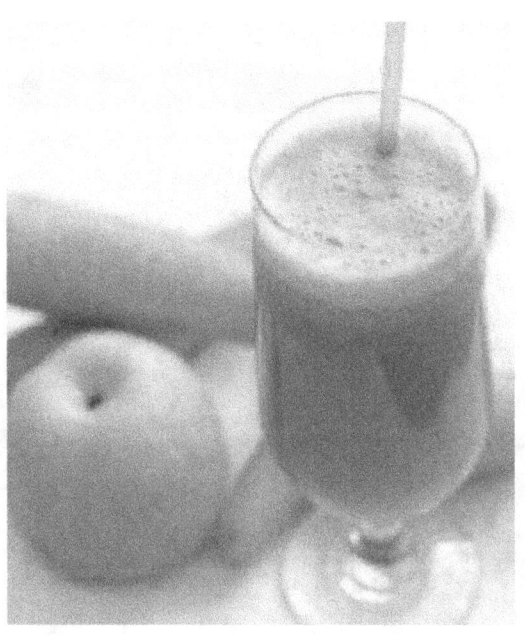

Nutritional Facts Per Serving:

Total Calories: 130

Fat: 0.75g

Protein: 2.28g

Carbohydrates: 40.87g

Fiber: 1.3g

Cholesterol: nil

Iron: 0.79mg

Sodium: 103mg

Calcium: 141mg

Carrot Juice with Fennel and Celery

For this juice, you will be needing two unpeeled carrots, one stalk of celery and half a cup of chopped fennel bulb. Before mixing all of these together, you would need to be sure that you clean all these vegetables. After cleaning, put the vegetables together in a juicer and enjoy.

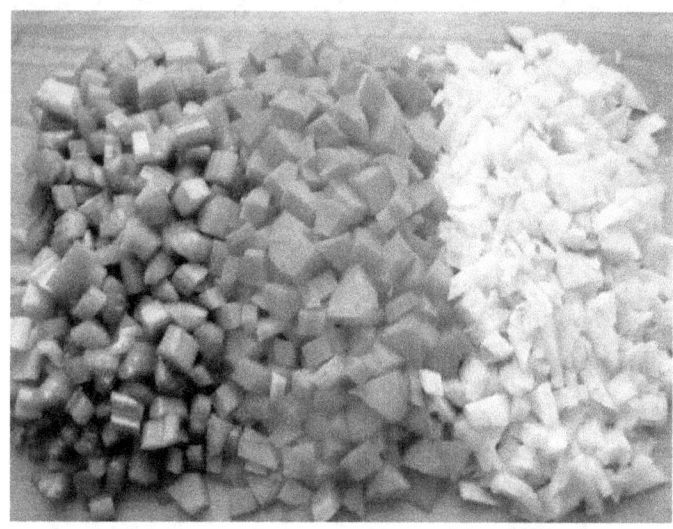

Nutritional Facts Per Serving:

Total Calories: 41

Fat: 0.36g

Protein: 1.67g

Carbohydrates: 13.38g

Fiber: 0.7g

Cholesterol: nil

Iron: 0.74mg

Sodium: 103mg

Calcium: 64mg

Carrot Mango Juice

The carrot mango juice consists of eight medium sized carrots, one pitted mango, one large orange peel strip, and half a peeled navel orange.

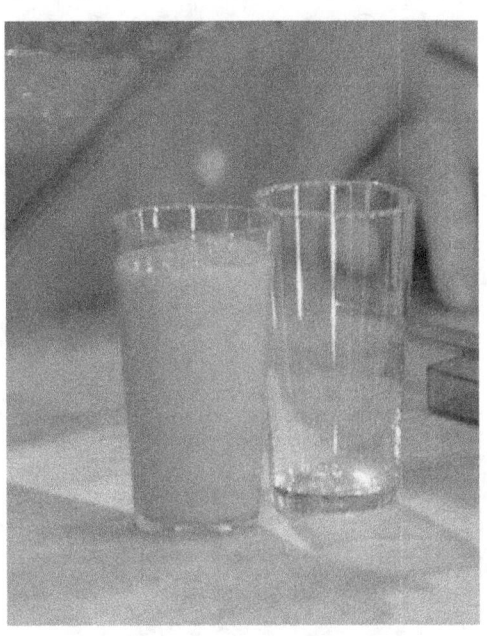

Nutritional Facts Per Serving:

Total Calories: 283

Fat: 1.87g

Protein: 6.32g

Carbohydrates: 83.09g

Fiber: 2.3g

Cholesterol: nil

Iron: 1.53mg

Sodium: 238mg

Calcium: 190mg

Cazapple Juice

Cazapple stands for carrot, zucchini and apple, and a mixture of these three ingredients forms a great juice with many health benefits which helps give you immense energy. To make this juice, you will be needing three large unpeeled carrots, two unpeeled and cored apples which are cut into slices, along with two medium unpeeled and quartered zucchini.

Make sure to wash these well before putting them in the juicer and enjoy the two servings worth of great taste.

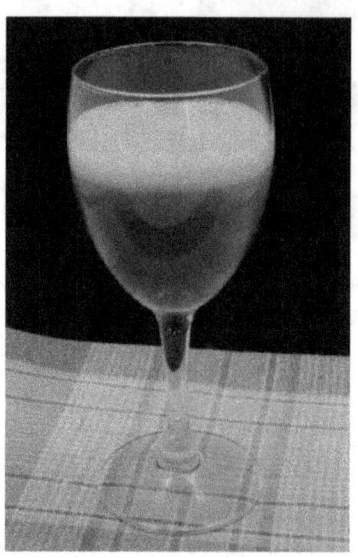

Nutritional Facts Per Serving:

Total Calories: 112

Fat: 0.91g

Protein: 2.86g

Carbohydrates: 34.01g

Fiber: 1.1g

Cholesterol: nil

Iron: 0.95mg

Sodium: 71mg

Calcium: 59mg

Creamy Mango Delight

The Creamy Mango Delight is just heaven and is perfect for beating the heat and relaxing. All you need to make this soothing drink is a half large and peeled mango, two unpeeled apples, half a cup of fresh pineapple cut into chunks and one unpeeled kiwifruit. This will give you one serving of juice.

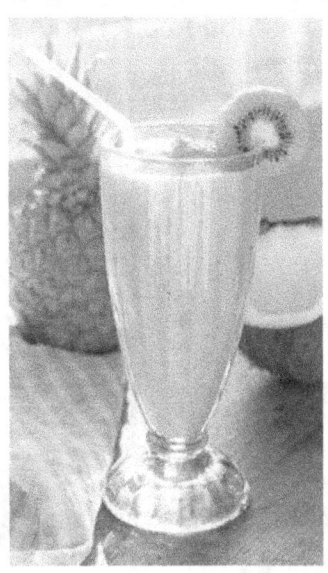

Nutritional Facts Per Serving:

Total Calories: 294

Fat: 1.64g

Protein: 3.65g

Carbohydrates: 86.27g

Fiber: 1.7g

Cholesterol: nil

Iron: 1.11mg

Sodium: 7mg

Calcium: 70mg

Detox

This Detox drink consists of high fiber root vegetables and ginger both of which have their own qualities. The root veggies for instance are great for your digestive track, while ginger works wonders for your stomach.

To make this drink, you would need two tablespoons of chopped and peeled fresh ginger, one medium chopped and scrubbed beet, four medium sliced and scrubbed carrots, one cubed and cored medium apple, and one cup water.

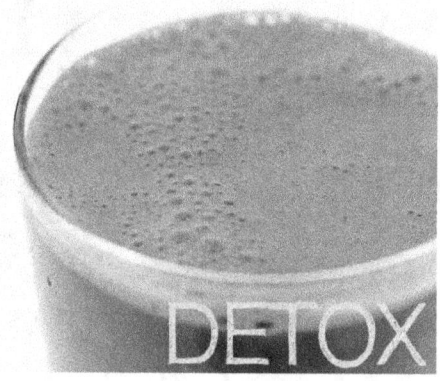

Nutritional Facts Per Serving:

Calories: 155

Fat: 0.7g

Protein: 3g

Carbohydrates: 37g

Fiber: 8g

Cholesterol: nil

Iron: 1mg

Sodium: 168mg

Calcium: 62mg

Energy Upper

This drink consists of coconut water and natural fruit sugars, both of which help to give you a boost in energy and keep you hydrated. All you need for this drink is one can of rinsed and drained lychees in syrup, one cup of thawed and frozen sliced peaches, and three fourth cup of either coconut water, or simply water.

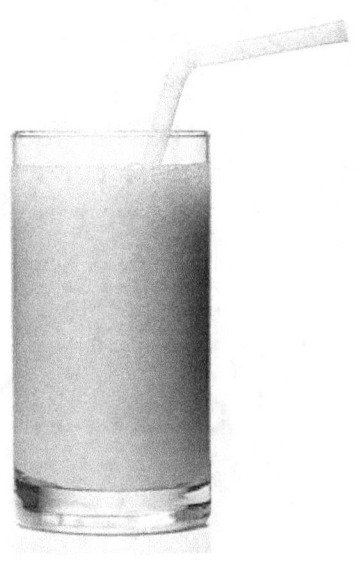

Nutritional Facts Per Serving:

Calories: 105

Fat: 0.6g

Protein: 2g

Carbohydrates: 26g

Fiber: 3g

Cholesterol: nil

Iron: 1mg

Sodium: 95mg

Calcium: 26mg

Everything Green

Ever since we were young, we had been told to consume green vegetables, and rightly so. Green foods consist of nutrients that help our overall bodily functions to perform in much better ways, and leave us healthier. The Everything Green juice incorporates the same healthy green vegetables and fruits to give you a better life.

In order to make the juice, you need two unpeeled Granny Smith apples which are cut into slices, one cup of fresh spinach with leaves intact, half of an unpeeled medium cucumber which should be about three inches long and cut in quarters lengthwise, one cup of green grapes, one fourth cup of packed parsley and half a lime at room temperature.

Remember to rinse well before mixing all these ingredients together. You will get two servings from the specified amount of ingredients.

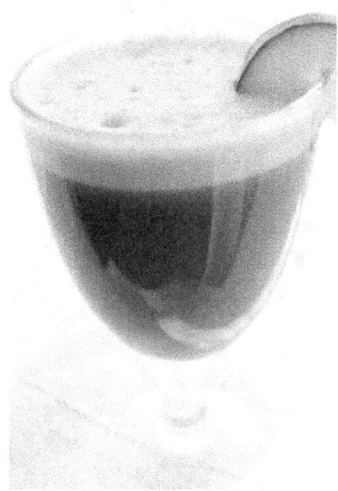

Nutritional Facts Per Serving:

Total Calories: 165

Fat: 1.28g

Protein: 4.18g

Carbohydrates: 52.71g

Fiber: 1.6g

Cholesterol: nil

Iron: 3.59mg

Sodium: 40mg

Calcium: 144mg

Fennel-Carrot Juice

Fennel is known to be slightly sweet and crunchy at the same time. It can be consumed cooked, raw or even as a juice. There are various health benefits of Fennel. It consists of vitamin C, is high in Fiber content, helps with amnesia, contains potassium, iron and folate and it helps soothes digestive problems.

In order to make a Fennel-Carrot juice, you need four to five large unpeeled carrots along with one fennel bulb with attached stalks. Wash well before juicing the produce so that you can thoroughly benefit from it. This will give you two servings.

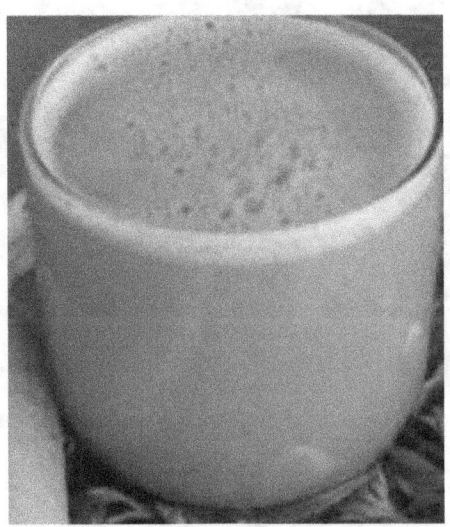

Nutritional Facts Per Serving:

Total Calories: 79

Fat: 0.69g

Protein: 3.44g

Carbohydrates: 26.44g

Fiber: 1.3g

Cholesterol: nil

Iron: 1.65mg

Sodium: 190mg

Calcium: 130mg

Garden Fresh Vegetable Juice

If you do not know much about juices, then you should know that this juice is not going to be sweet, nor would it tastes as yummy as the rest of the fruit juices. However, this juice will provide you with many benefits and nutrients that your body needs.

You would require three ripe tomatoes, two cups of fresh spinach leaves, two stalks of celery, one cup of chopped red cabbage, six basil leaves and one fourth cup of fresh lightly packed parsley.

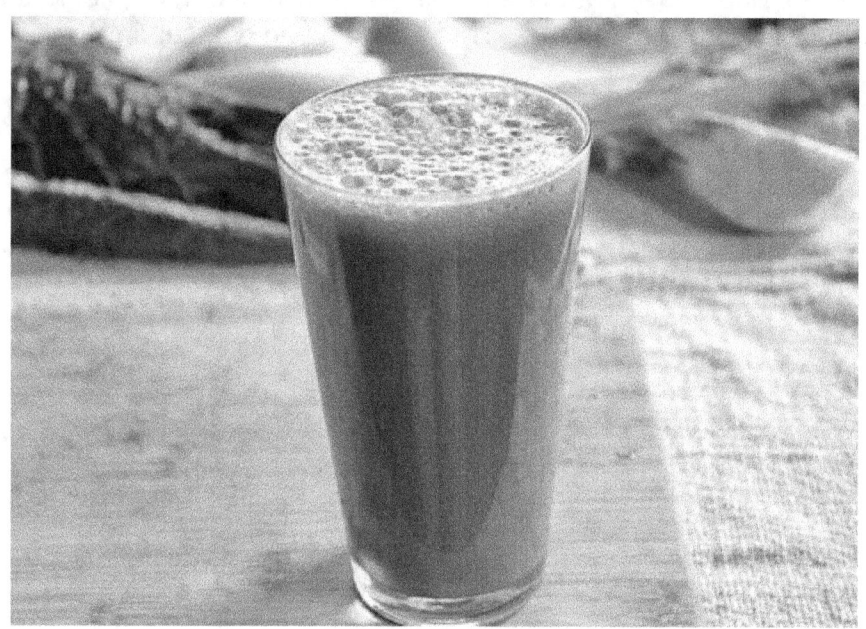

Nutritional Facts Per Serving:

Total Calories: 58

Fat: 0.97g

Protein: 5.10g

Carbohydrates: 16.31g

Fiber: 0.9g

Cholesterol: nil

Iron: 4.27mg

Sodium: 95mg

Calcium: 155mg

Garden Green Coco

Coconuts have electrolytes and potassium which make the drink great post workout and for the summer season. To make this drink you would need one Thai coconut, one handful of green kale, one handful of spinach, and half a banana.

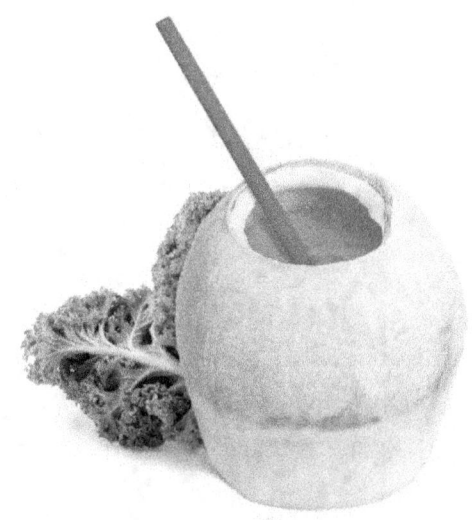

Nutritional Facts Per Serving:

Total Calories: 941

Fat: 93.50g

Protein: 11.25g

Carbohydrates: 54.54g

Fiber: 4g

Cholesterol: nil

Iron: 7.69 mg

Sodium: 79mg

Calcium: 95mg

Grapefruit Carrot and Ginger Juice

This drink has immune boosting capabilities and a lot of fiber for your body to function normally. You can prepare this juice easily with two chopped and peeled grapefruits, five chopped carrots and one inch of peeled chopped and fresh ginger.

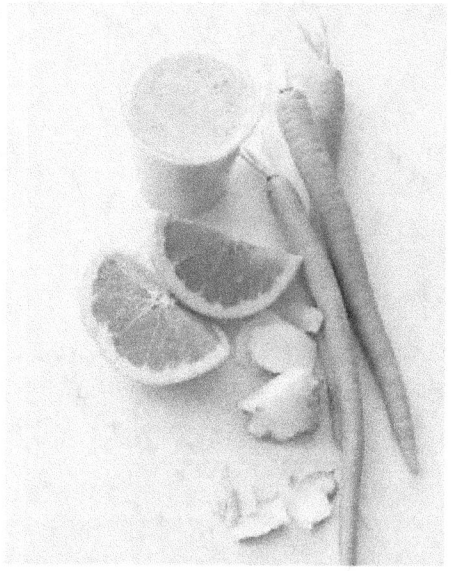

Nutritional Facts Per Serving:

Total Calories: 145

Fat: 0.83g

Protein: 3.70 g

Carbohydrates: 42.37g

Fiber: 1.2g

Cholesterol: nil

Iron: 0.88mg

Sodium: 123mg

Calcium: 94mg

Green Juice

The Green Juice is an amazing, refreshing and a healthy drink consisting of veggies and apples for taste. You can adjust the vegetable and fruit amounts according to your taste. To make this drink, you will be requiring two green apples, six kale leaves, four celery stalks with leaves removed, half a peeled lemon, one cucumber, and one (one-inch) piece of fresh ginger. This combination will give you a serving size of two people.

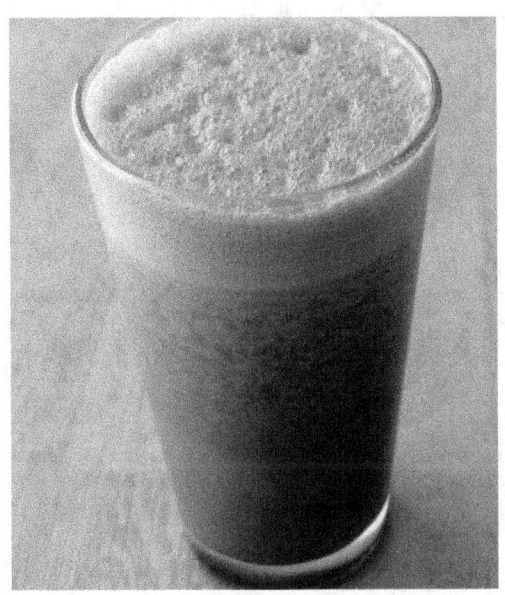

Nutritional Facts Per Serving:

Total Calories: 106

Fat: 1.11g

Protein: 4.53g

Carbohydrates: 27.80g

Fiber: 0.6g

Cholesterol: nil

Iron: 1.66mg

Sodium: 51mg

Calcium: 147mg

Hello Sunshine Orange Juice

This Hello Sunshine Orange juice consists of apples, oranges, and red seedless grapes to make a perfect drink resembling pure sunshine and brightness.

Take two peeled oranges and divide them into segments, two unpeeled apples which are cut into slices (discard the cores), and one cup of red seedless grapes. Mix these fruits well in the juicer and your serving for two is ready.

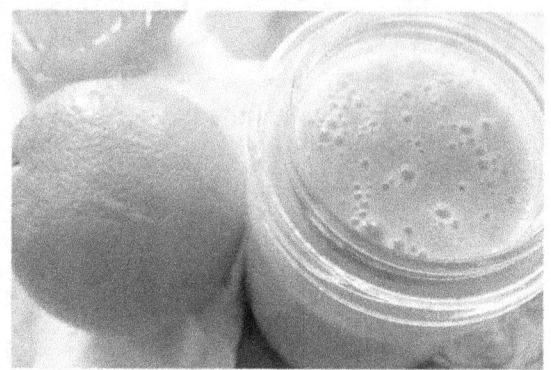

Nutritional Facts Per Serving:

Total Calories: 107

Fat: 0.58g

Protein: 1.64g

Carbohydrates: 33.95g

Fiber: 1.0g

Cholesterol: nil

Iron: 0.38mg

Sodium: 2mg

Calcium: 66mg

Immune Booster

The Immune Booster helps to boost your immune system, and as a result keeps you protects from colds and other common illnesses. The Kiwis in the drink contain a lot of vitamin C, while oranges fight off your cold in an instant.

You can easily make this fighter drink by getting one peeled grapefruit, two medium peeled oranges, and three peeled kiwis.

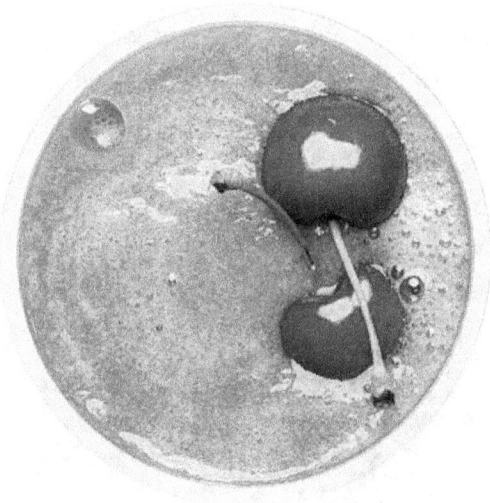

Nutritional Facts:

Calories: 156

Fat: 1g

Protein: 3g

Carbohydrates: 38g

Fiber: 6g

Cholesterol: nil

Iron: 1mg

Sodium: 5 mg

Calcium: 79mg

Kale-Orange Juice

Oranges are great for you, and an orange partnered with kale is the greatest combination of all. Kale is high in vitamin C, A and K, consists of omega-3 fatty acids and fiber, along with being a great antioxidant. That is great for just one vegetable.

To make the Kale-Orange juice, you would be needing three large peeled navel oranges and two cups of chopped kale leaves with ribs removed.

Make sure that you wash the kale leaves well after which you can put these ingredients in the juicer to prepare two servings worth of juice.

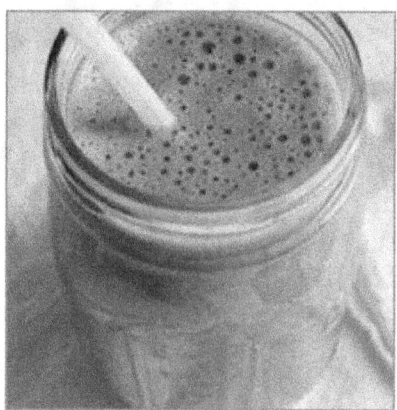

Nutritional Facts Per Serving:

Total Calories: 110

Fat: 0.92g

Protein: 4.96 g

Carbohydrates: 29.13g

Fiber: 1g

Cholesterol: nil

Iron: 1.27mg

Sodium: 28mg

Calcium: 188mg

New York-Style Fennel Juice

This New York-Style Fennel Juice consists of carrots, tomatoes, fennel bulb, and fresh parsley. In order to make two servings, you would be needing two unpeeled carrots with tops removed, two quartered tomatoes, half sliced fennel bulb, and one fourth packed fresh parsley. The juice will be so refreshing that your entire day will brighten up automatically.

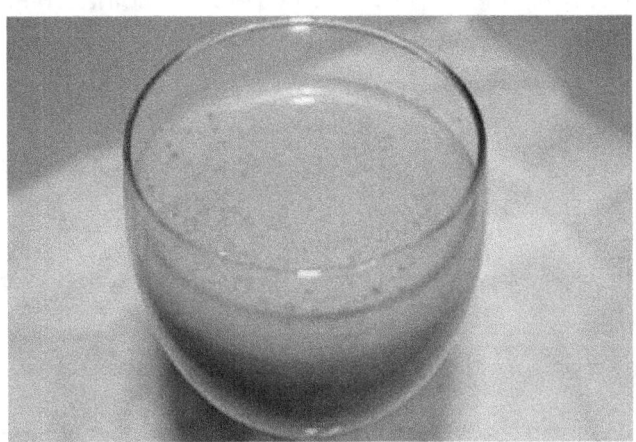

Nutritional Facts Per Serving:

Total Calories: 45

Fat: 0.61g

Protein: 2.80g

Carbohydrates: 14.32g

Fiber: 0.8g

Cholesterol: nil

Iron: 2.63mg

Sodium: 91mg

Calcium: 99mg

Orange, Blueberry & Spinach Twist

Orange, blueberry, and spinach twist is an amazing juice, especially post workout. If you are a little worried about how the spinach is going to taste, you should know that the spinach taste is completely masked with the help of orange and blueberry.

The juice can be made with two large and peeled oranges divided into segments, one cup of fresh blueberries, and one cup of freshly packed spinach leaves. This will give you a serving size of two people.

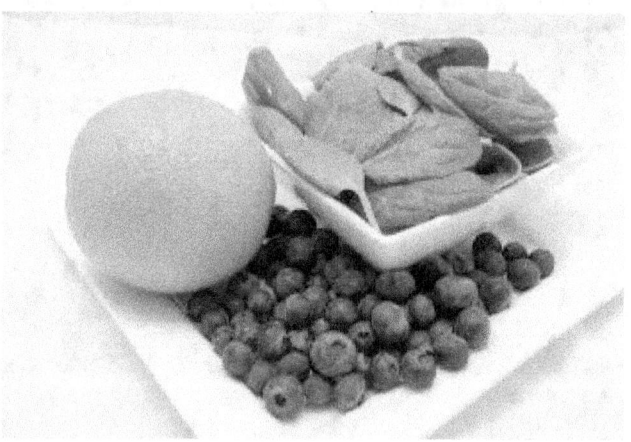

Nutritional Facts Per Serving:

Total Calories: 76

Fat: 0.37g

Protein: 1.89g

Carbohydrates: 23.02g

Fiber: 0.7g

Cholesterol: nil

Iron: 0.56mg

Sodium: 9mg

Calcium: 65mg

Orange-Carrot Juice

This amazing and healthy orange carrot juice can be made from two large peeled oranges and three unpeeled carrots with their tops removed. The juice, once made can be given to two people who will feel refreshing after having it.

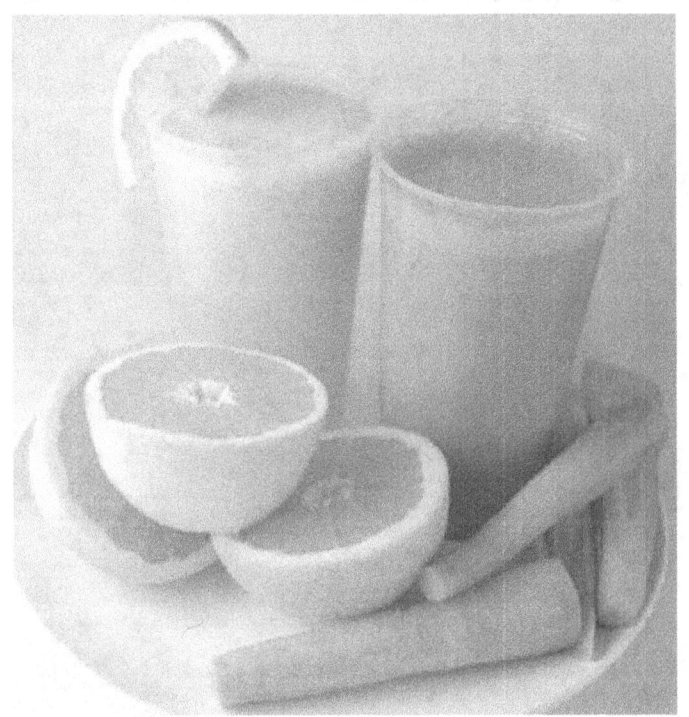

Nutritional Facts Per Serving:

Total Calories: 66

Fat: 0.28g

Protein: 1.70g

Carbohydrates: 20.16g

Fiber: 0.7g

Cholesterol: nil

Iron: 0.29mg

Sodium: 36mg

Calcium: 69mg

Orient Express

This juice consists of fresh ginger root amongst other things, which is great for reducing motion sickness, alleviating nausea, having anti-inflammatory properties, and soothing gastrointestinal distress. When you buy fresh ginger root, be sure to refrigerate it so that its freshness can last a long time. In order to make this juice, you need three unpeeled carrots with tops removed, two large unpeeled apples, and one unpeeled slice of ginger root.

Nutritional Facts Per Serving:

Total Calories: 96

Fat: 0.52g

Protein: 1.20g

Carbohydrates: 29.57g

Fiber: 0.8g

Cholesterol: nil

Iron: 0.45mg

Sodium: 40mg

Calcium: 29mg

Pineapple Papaya Juice

This juice is healthy, refreshing and a great start to your new day. The drink can be made from five sprigs of fresh mint, one peeled pineapple cut into pieces, and one medium peeled and seeded papaya.

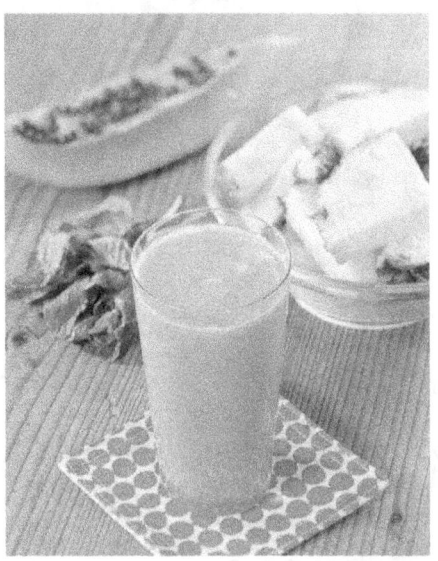

Nutritional Facts Per Serving:

Total Calories: 325

Fat: 1.05g

Protein: 3.94g

Carbohydrates: 95.01g

Fiber: 1.5g

Cholesterol: nil

Iron: 2.11mg

Sodium: 15mg

Calcium: 104mg

Pomegranate Citrus Juice

The juice can be made with two small grapefruits, two oranges, two mineola tangelos or tangerines, half lime and two pomegranates. The drink is refreshing, great for your body, and full of color and antioxidants.

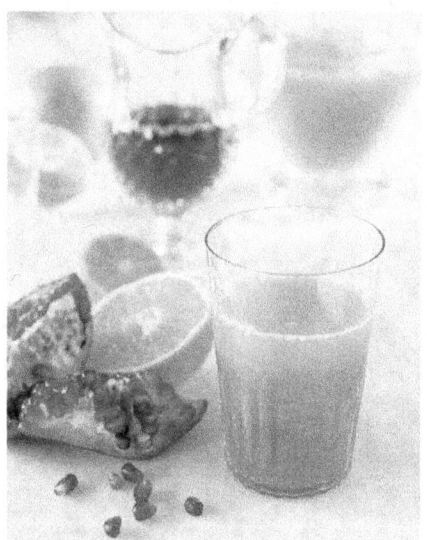

Nutritional Facts Per Serving:

Total Calories: 411

Fat: 5.33g

Protein: 9.52g

Carbohydrates: 115.36g

Fiber: 3.1g

Cholesterol: nil

Iron: 1.76mg

Sodium: 15mg

Calcium: 126mg

Post Workout Refueler

This rejuvenating juice consists of almonds, oranges, sweet potato, and apple. Therefore, a combination such as this gives you adequate amount of protein required for muscle building and repair, along with potassium required to balance fluids and electrolytes.

In order to make the drink, you would need two medium sized peeled oranges, one fourth cup of raw almonds, one small scrubbed sweet potato, one medium apple, and half a cup of water.

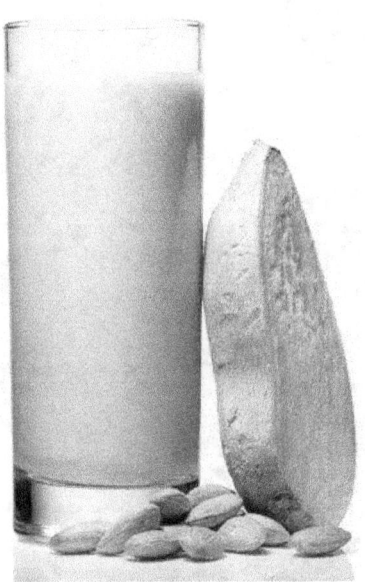

Nutritional Facts Per Serving:

Total Calories: 231

Fat: 9.1g

Protein: 6g

Carbohydrates: 36g

Fiber: 7g

Cholesterol: nil

Iron: 1mg

Sodium: 24mg

Calcium: 106mg

Potassium Broth

Potassium Broth consists of potassium which is beneficial for your body and for regenerating your cells. It also helps to reduce stomach acidity and the celery and parsley in the juice helps prevent cancer. To make the juice you would need three to five carrots, three to four celery stalks, a handful of spinach, and a handful of parsley.

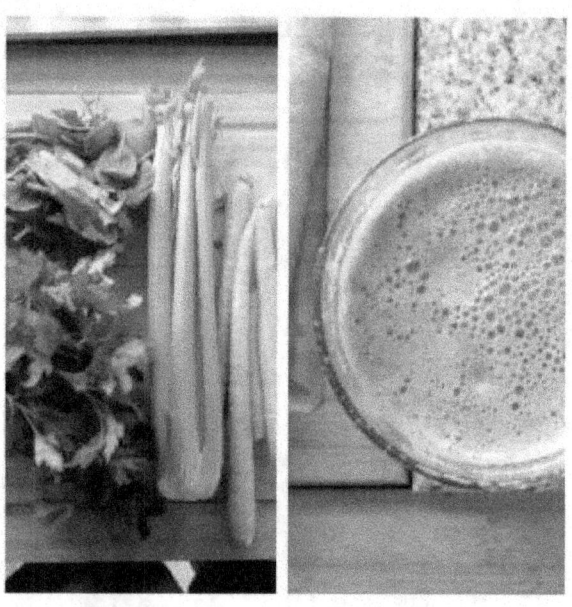

Nutritional Facts Per Serving:

Total Calories: 56

Fat: 0.69g

Protein: 2.88g

Carbohydrates: 16.88g

Fiber: 0.8g

Cholesterol: nil

Iron: 2.70mg

Sodium: 155mg

Calcium: 116mg

Power Gulp

This green energy drink is filled with iron, which is extra beneficial during pregnancy and menstruation. Iron also helps in proper functioning of your muscles and healthy blood cells. Another great feature of this drink is that you receive sufficient vitamin K which is beneficial for your bone and blood health.

To make this drink you will need one cup of sliced kale, one cup of green seedless grapes, one English and thickly sliced cucumber, one small Granny Smith apple, and about half a cup of water.

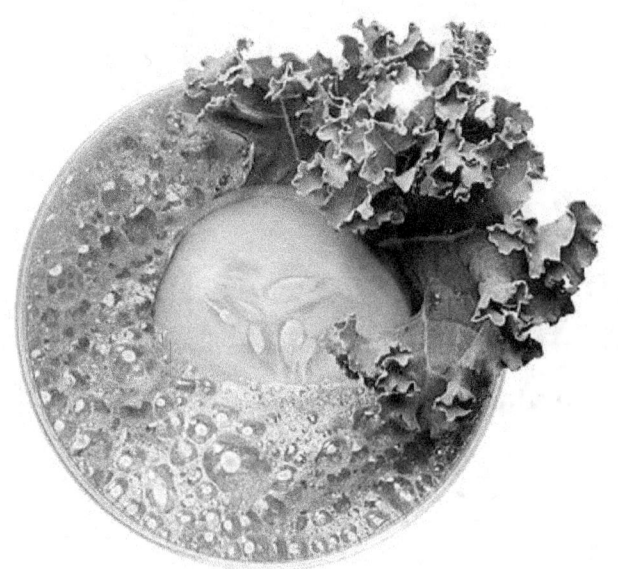

Nutritional Facts Per Serving:

Total Calories: 110

Fat: 0.6g

Protein: 3g

Carbohydrates: 27g

Fiber: 3g

Cholesterol: nil

Iron: 1mg

Sodium: 19mg

Calcium: 77mg

Refreshing Romaine Salad...in a Glass

This refreshing romaine salad in a glass is made from one cup torn romaine packed lettuce, half a cup broccoli florets, two unpeeled apples, and one orange which will give you two energy packed servings. Take care to put the broccoli and the lettuce along with the fruit in the juicer so that they mix and juice well.

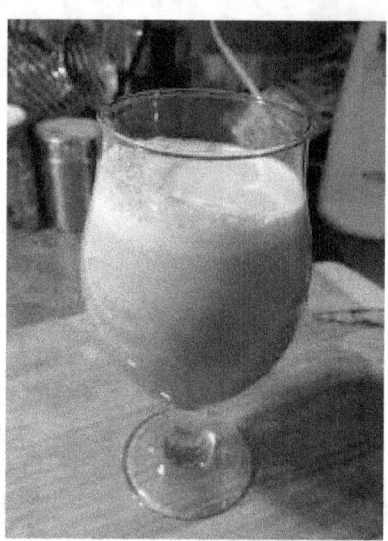

Nutritional Facts Per Serving:

Total Calories: 65

Fat: 0.29g

Protein: 0.96g

Carbohydrates: 20.46g

Fiber: 0.6g

Cholesterol: nil

Iron: 0.34mg

Sodium: 3mg

Calcium: 31mg

Ruby Red Beet Juice

The Ruby Red Beet Juice consists of one beet with its ends removed, two peeled oranges divided into segments, and two unpeeled apples which are cut into slices.

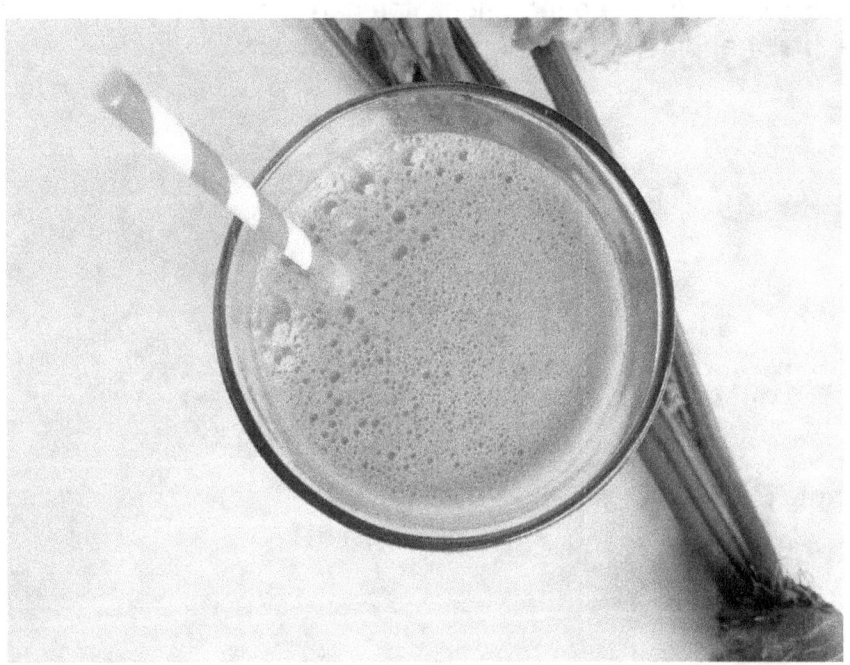

Nutritional Facts Per Serving:

Total Calories: 201

Fat: 0.78g

Protein: 4.24g

Carbohydrates: 62.07g

Fiber: 1.8g

Cholesterol: nil

Iron: 1.41mg

Sodium: 98mg

Calcium: 105mg

Savage Cabbage Juice

A mix of cabbage, parsley, and carrots will give you a drink that is highly beneficial for you. The drink is great for the immune system, eyes, and skin, and helps to prevent stroke, cataracts, or macular degeneration. You can prepare this drink with half medium head cabbage, half handful parsley, and four medium sized carrots.

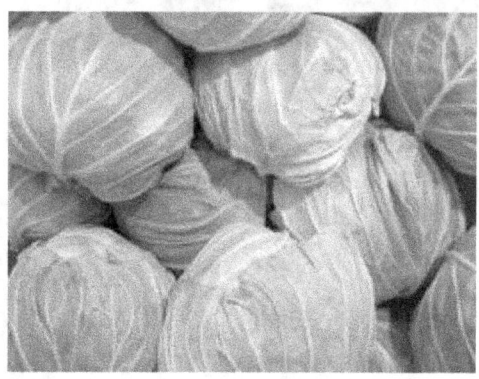

Nutritional Facts Per Serving:

Total Calories: 107

Fat: 0.84g

Protein: 6.07g

Carbohydrates: 35.68g

Fiber: 1.9g

Cholesterol: nil

Iron: 2.87mg

Sodium: 183mg

Calcium: 203mg

South Pacific Sunrise

This amazing juice has been inspired by New Zealand and can be made from two unpeeled and cored Fuji or Gala apples, two large unpeeled carrots, two unpeeled, and halved kiwifruit and two cups of packed spinach. The greens are always easier to juice when combined with other vegetables or fruits.

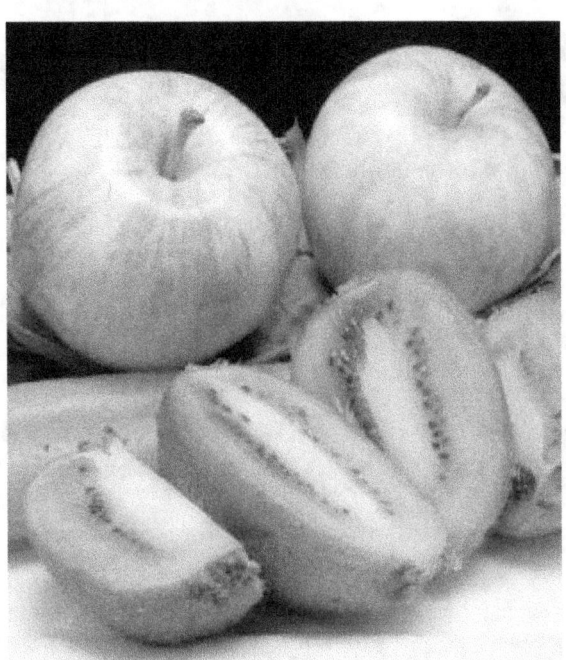

Nutritional Facts Per Serving:

Total Calories: 129

Fat: 0.84g

Protein: 3.86g

Carbohydrates: 38.76g

Fiber: 1.3g

Cholesterol: nil

Iron: 1.98mg

Sodium: 149mg

Calcium: 80mg

Spinach Cucumber Celery Juice

This juice is great for your body since it helps eliminate toxins from your body, improves the overall immune system, consists of anti-inflammatory properties, and helps to purify the blood. In order to make this juice you will need to mix together two cups of packed spinach, one cucumber and one celery stalk.

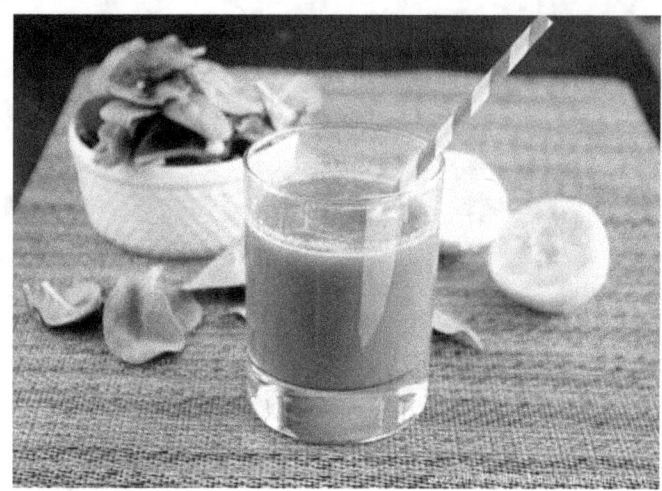

Nutritional Facts Per Serving:

Total Calories: 35

Fat: 0.42g

Protein: 2.65g

Carbohydrates: 9.57g

Fiber: 0.3g

Cholesterol: nil

Iron: 1.75mg

Sodium: 47mg

Calcium: 80mg

Strawberry Hill Juice

This juice is fresh and minty which helps to prevent osteoporosis along with cancer while at the same time giving you a lot of energy and boosting your immune system. to make this juice you will be needing one cup of whole strawberries, one medium pear, a half of pineapple and around fifteen peppermint leaves.

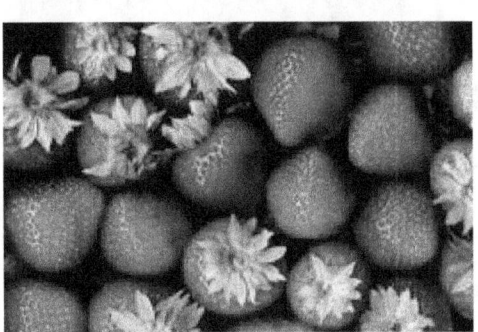

Nutritional Facts Per Serving:

Total Calories: 225

Fat: 0.87g

Protein: 2.87g

Carbohydrates: 68.43g

Fiber: 1.5g

Cholesterol: nil

Iron: 1.61mg

Sodium: 6mg

Calcium: 71mg

Sweet Licorice Juice

This drink consists of one fourth pineapple, half fennel bulb, and about seven carrots. The pineapple and the carrots help to make the licorice taste much more pleasant.

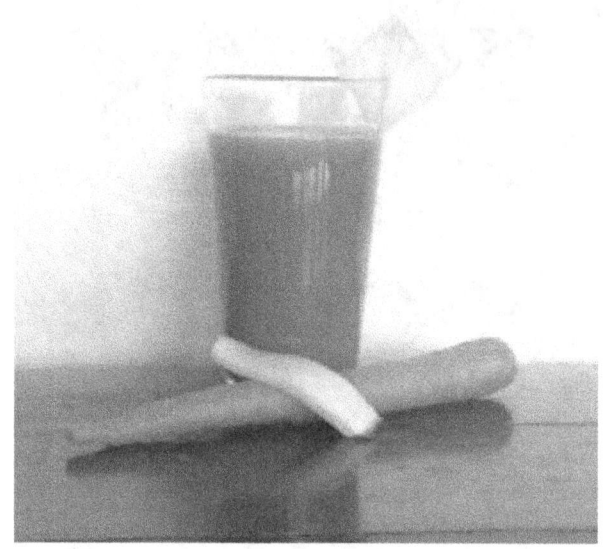

Nutritional Facts Per Serving:

Total Calories: 163

Fat: 0.94g

Protein: 4.15g

Carbohydrates: 50.23g

Fiber: 1.7g

Cholesterol: nil

Iron: 1.79mg

Sodium: 213mg

Calcium: 142mg

Tangy Apple Delight

The tangy mango delight will give you the benefit of three amazing fruits, apples, grapefruit, and grapes. To make the juice, you will need to mix together two unpeeled apples, one peeled grapefruit, and one cup of red seedless grapes in a juicer.

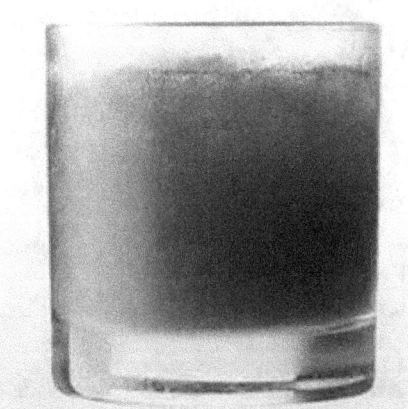

Nutritional Facts Per Serving:

Total Calories: 84

Fat: 0.41g

Protein: 1.09g

Carbohydrates: 26.03g

Fiber: 0.7g

Cholesterol: nil

Iron: 0.29mg

Sodium: 1mg

Calcium: 29mg

The Ginger Zinger

This juice contains ingredients and antioxidants necessary for good health and strength. It helps to remove toxins from your system, and activate you metabolism. To make this juice, you will need two apples, two carrots, one slice of lemon, and one forth inch of ginger along with ice cubes.

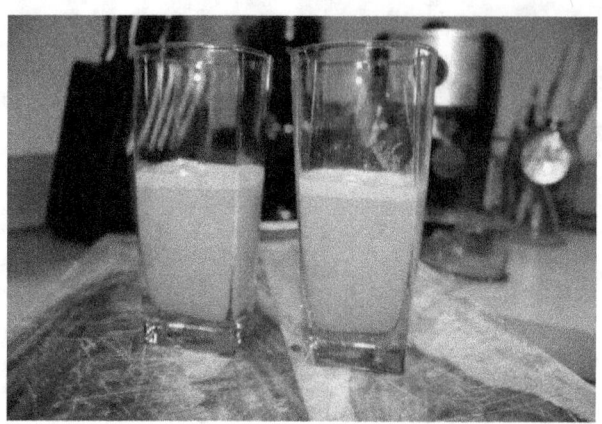

Nutritional Facts Per Serving:

Total Calories: 121

Fat: 0.61g

Protein: 1.47g

Carbohydrates: 38.19g

Fiber: 1.1g

Cholesterol: nil

Iron: 0.56mg

Sodium: 62mg

Calcium: 43mg

The Hot 'n' Spicy

This drink is perfect for maintaining good health, and helps flush out your kidneys and liver, for a hydrated and fresh looking skin. To make this drink you need three apples and a pinch of cinnamon.

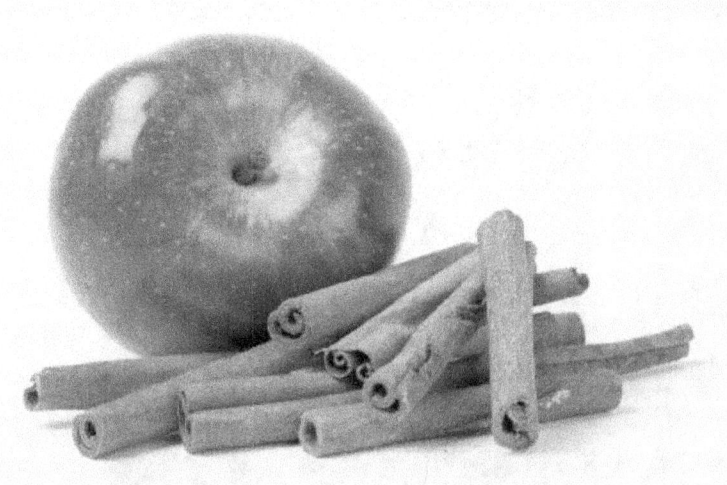

Nutritional Facts Per Serving:

Total Calories: 136

Fat: 0.54g

Protein: 0.83g

Carbohydrates: 43.58g

Fiber: 1.1g

Cholesterol: nil

Iron: 0.41mg

Sodium: 3mg

Calcium: 23mg

The Iron Man

A lot of people are deficient in iron, which is why this is one of the most important minerals that one should strive to get. Iron helps with your concentration, and is great for your nails and hair. This juice also consists of calcium, which is good for bones and teeth. To make this drink you would require one apple, one forth pineapple, one forth banana, 200g soya, and half teaspoon of spirulina.

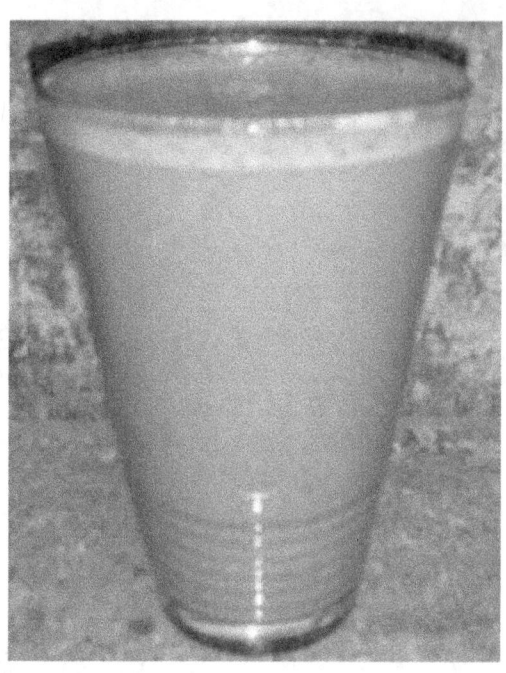

Nutritional Facts Per Serving:

Total Calories: 142

Fat: 0.91g

Protein: 2.62g

Carbohydrates: 40.68g

Fiber: 0.8g

Cholesterol: nil

Iron: 1mg

Sodium: 12mg

Calcium: 33mg

The Minty Beta

This juice mainly consists of carrots, which are rich in beta-carotene. This beta-carotene is a powerful antioxidant known to prevent cancer, and also helps with digestion, cleanser the liver, and reduces cholesterol. For this drink, you will need four carrots, a handful of diced mint leaves, and half a teaspoon of spirulina.

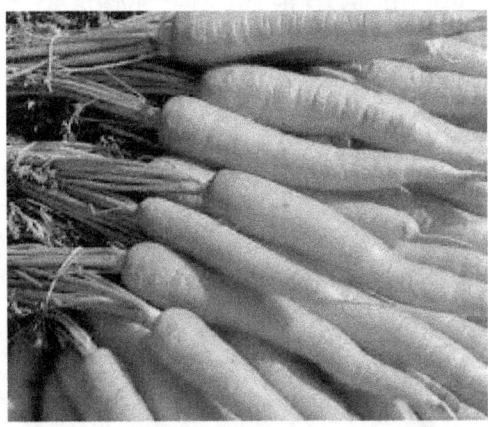

Nutritional Facts Per Serving:

Total Calories: 55

Fat: 0.47g

Protein: 2.06g

Carbohydrates: 16.58g

Fiber: 0.7g

Cholesterol: nil

Iron: 0.75mg

Sodium: 126mg

Calcium: 58mg

The Turbo Express

You can help to boost your immune system with this drink. Being rich in vitamin C, iron, potassium, protein, and natural sugars, the juice is also great for your red blood cells and white blood cells. To make this delicious and healthy juice you would require two apples, one handful of spinach leaves, one slice of cucumber, one slice of lime, half a stick of celery, one quarter pineapple, one quarter avocado, and ice cubes to make a chilled refreshing drink.

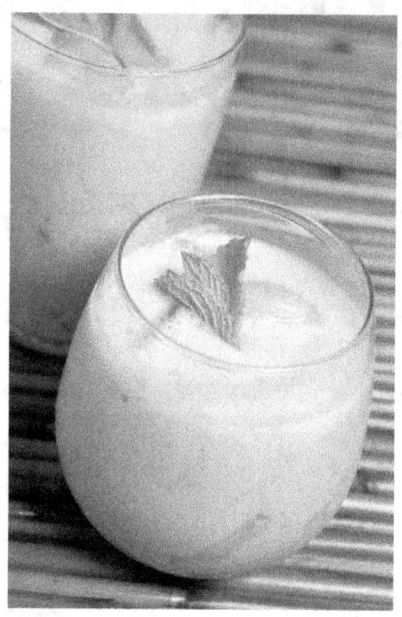

Nutritional Facts Per Serving:

Total Calories: 270

Fat: 6.18g

Protein: 4.46g

Carbohydrates: 72.37g

Fiber: 1.9g

Cholesterol: nil

Iron: 2.32mg

Sodium: 30mg

Calcium: 109mg

Tomato Juice

Tomato juice will consists of two large quartered tomatoes, two unpeeled carrots with tops removed, and two stalks of celery with their tops included.

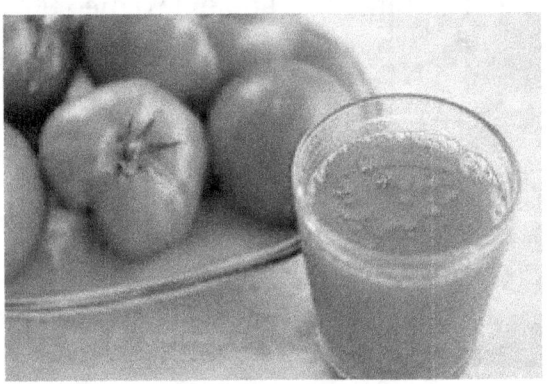

Nutritional Facts Per Serving:

Total Calories: 29

Fat: 0.36g

Protein: 1.53g

Carbohydrates: 8.66g

Fiber: 0.4g

Cholesterol: nil

Iron: 0.47mg

Sodium: 40mg

Calcium: 29mg

Total Health Booster

This juice is packed with vitamins A, B, C, and E along with Lutein, which helps to fight aging because it facilitates collagen production for healthy skin and stronger bones. The drink can be made from one medium sized apple, two medium soft pears like Bartlett, and half a cup of fresh cherries.

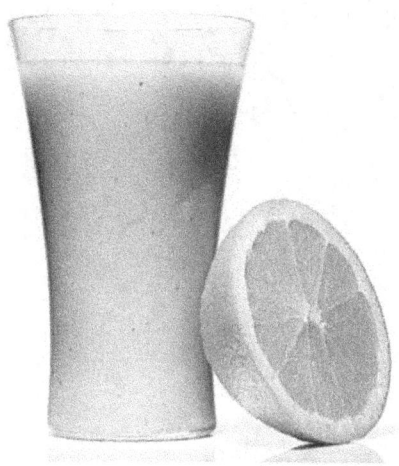

Nutritional Facts Per Serving:

Total Calories: 192

Fat: 0.4g

Protein: 1g

Carbohydrates: 51g

Fiber: 8g

Cholesterol: nil

Iron: 1mg

Sodium: 2mg

Calcium: 29mg

Tropical Paradise Juice

This juice will brighten up your day and give you a fresh start. It helps clear out any buildup you might have while you were sleeping, and helps to hydrate your body. To make this juice you will need one medium peeled, seeded, and sliced ripe papaya, one small peeled, sliced, and cored pineapple, one peeled fresh ginger, one medium and peeled kiwi, along with one and a half cup of fresh coconut water.

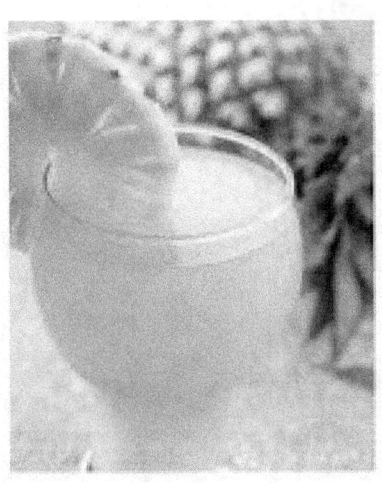

Nutritional Facts Per Serving:

Total Calories: 90

Fat: 0.87g

Protein: 2.28g

Carbohydrates: 25.20g

Fiber: 0.7g

Cholesterol: nil

Iron: 0.91mg

Sodium: 187mg

Calcium: 79mg

Tropical Tango

This beneficial drink consists of two medium sized peaches with pits removed, two medium pears, and a half pineapple fruit. The drink helps to prevent osteoporosis, reduce inflammation, strengthen the immune system, and prevent cancer.

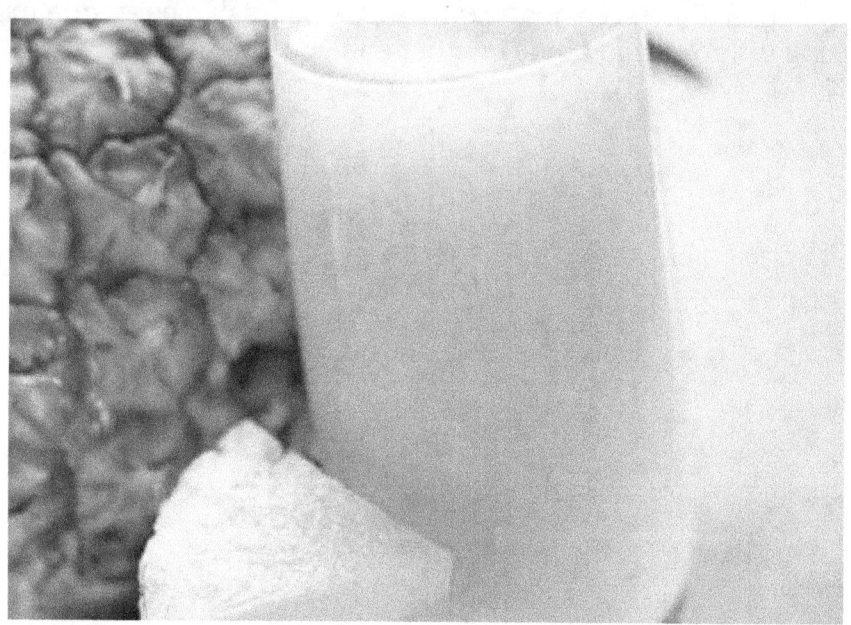

Nutritional Facts Per Serving:

Total Calories: 327

Fat: 1.25g

Protein: 4.52g

Carbohydrates: 99.54g

Fiber: 2.2g

Cholesterol: nil

Iron: 1.89mg

Sodium: 6mg

Calcium: 76mg

Wild Spiced Dandelion Berry Bliss Juice

The Wild Spiced Dandelion Berry Bliss Juice is a one of a kind drink which will refresh you completely from within. It is pleasing, healthy, and consists of some of the most amazing fruits. To make this drink, you will be required to mix together two cups of strawberries, one cup of dandelion leaves to add taste, one cup of raspberries, and one small chili with removes placental skin and seeds.

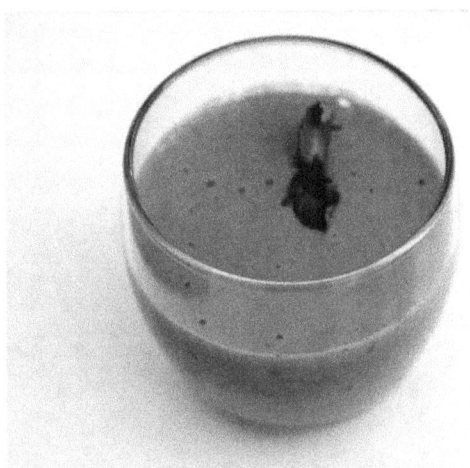

Nutritional Facts Per Serving:

Total Calories: 98

Fat: 1.57g

Protein: 4.01g

Carbohydrates: 32.08g

Fiber: 1.6g

Cholesterol: nil

Iron: 2.94mg

Sodium: 35mg

Calcium: 130mg